Stress, Anxiety, Solutions

John Harriyott

DEDICATION

To all who suffer anxiety and related stresses, may
this book bring some hope for a better future.

CONTENTS

PROLOGUE

Do you want to reduce your stress levels?

Yes... Are you sure?

Yes..Yes. Yes!

Good then this is the book to help you do just that.

The main causes of stress are individually dealt with in separate chapters, complete with practical day to day ways of working to eliminate them from your life.

We cover how to initially manage stress.
Then how to deal with mental, physical, emotional and psychological stress.

The aim is to bring your stress and anxiety levels back down a state of relaxation.
Come and join me.

1 ABOUT STRESS

What is stress?

Stress is the feeling of being under too much mental or emotional pressure.

Pressure turns into stress when you feel unable to cope. People have different ways of reacting to stress, so a situation that feels stressful to one person may be motivating to someone else.

Many of many of the things we do every day can cause stress, particularly work, relationships and money problems.

And, when you feel stressed, it can get in the way of sorting out these demands, or can even affect everything you do.

Stress can affect how you feel, think, behave and how your body works. In fact, common signs of stress include sleeping problems, sweating, loss of appetite and difficulty concentrating.

You may feel anxious, irritable or low in self esteem, and you may have racing thoughts, worry constantly or go over things in your head.

You may notice that you lose your temper more easily (yes I know, but we do get to the solutions very soon), drink more or act unreasonably.

You may also experience headaches, muscle tension or pain, or dizziness.

Stress causes a surge of hormones in your body. These stress hormones are released to enable you to deal with pressures or threats – the so-called "fight or flight" response.

Once the pressure or threat has passed, your stress hormone levels will usually return to normal.

However, if you're constantly under stress, these hormones will remain in your body, leading to the symptoms of stress.

But stress comes from many differing causes and we will be looking at three that are the cause many problems.

MENTAL: worry, anxiety, perfectionism, long work hours

PHYSICAL: lack of sleep, travel, manual labour.

EMOTIONAL: loneliness, sadness, guilt, anger, fear, financial

So are you Stressed?
Here are some Signs and Symptoms of Stress:

Emotional

Moodiness

Irritability or short temper

Agitation, inability to relax

Feeling overwhelmed

Sense of loneliness and isolation

Depression or general unhappiness

Behavioural

Eating more or less

Sleeping too much or too little

Isolating yourself from others

Procrastinating or neglecting responsibilities

Using alcohol, cigarettes, or drugs to relax

Nervous habits (e.g. nail biting, pacing)

Physical

Aches and pains

Diarrhoea or constipation

Nausea, dizziness

Chest pain, rapid heartbeat

Loss of sex drive

Frequent colds

Cognitive

Memory problems

Inability to concentrate

Poor judgement

Seeing only the negative

Anxious or racing thoughts

Constant worrying

2 DEALING WITH STRESS

Always remember this very important truism:

If there is something (anything) that is upsetting you, do something about it.

If there really is nothing <u>YOU</u> can do about it, accept it and get on with the rest your life.

3   HOW TO MANAGE STRESS

Laughter is one of the healthiest antidotes to stress. When we laugh or even smile, blood flow to the brain is increased, endorphins (painkilling hormones that give us a sense of well being) are released, and levels of stress hormones drop.

There are plenty of other effective (and mostly pleasant) things you can do to minimize and manage stress.

"Instant" stress relief

But before we get into too much detail on long term solutions I want to show you some instant stress relieving solutions. They have a well known group name of relaxation.

We have all heard people say just relax, but they seldom explain how to relax, so here we go.

Relaxation, how to use it to reduce your stress levels.

Do this before reading any more chapters.

The easiest way to relax is to sit in a chair (or on the floor) and put your hands in your lap.
Then look at your hands and also feel your chest breathing in and out.

Concentrate on this and as you breath in and out, say to yourself - breath in, breath out.
Try to concentrate just on that, let all other thoughts drift by, and gradually slow down your breathing.

To start with it will be difficult to let go of all the pressing worries and thoughts charging into your mind but the more you concentrate on the breathing and allow all other thoughts to slip by, the easier it will get.

Do this for about five minutes.

Whilst this will give you instant relief, it may take up to 3 weeks before it seems to come naturally and work without any effort.

Indeed you will find that if you do this at the start of the day it will boost your ability to face the world.

Another very good time to relax is as you get into

bed.

Lay flat on your back, hands by your side.
Squeeze up your toes as tight as you can hold it like that for about 2 seconds then let them go.
Next do the same thing with your calf muscles, squeeze, hold, let go.
Next same again with the thighs,
Then the chest,
After that clench your hands, squeeze, hold, let go.
Now the same with your arms.
Finally, clamp your teeth tight together, hold for 2 seconds and then un-clamp.

What you have done is to allow each part of your body to relax, so keep that relaxed state, try not to dwell on any one thought that enters your mind, just drift off to sleep.

Final thought on relaxing is something you can do any time of the day.

It is to simply drop your shoulders.

For as we tense up our shoulders rise, so as soon as you realise what you are doing just un-tension yourself by letting your shoulders drop down.

Sure, within a minute or two they may tense up and you will need to do it again. This if nothing else will highlight that you are under stress, so look around, what is the current situation that is causing your shoulders to rise up?

4 WHAT TYPE OF STRESS DO YOU HAVE

I doubt if any of us have just one simple specific cause that makes us stressful, so let's first seek out the area that is having the greatest pull.

As each day develops and stress mounts up, write down the when, why and how as soon as the stress starts, if not immediately then as soon as practical afterwards.

What we are trying to do is find a pattern. It may be blatantly obvious to you like you're flat broke and get stressed every time a letter drops through the letterbox. However often it is deeper than that.

So start collecting this vital 'intelligence'.

At the end of each day run through the 5 minute relaxation exercise then study your notes and put them into some sort of order, then after a few days a broad pattern may start to appear.

You may find in broad terms that travelling to work, speaking to a certain person, hot/cold environment, a certain time of day etc. stands out as a possible reason.

Compare these possible reasons with the signs and symptoms shown earlier.
Work on this until you feel you have a good indication as to the trigger points that stress you out.

Once at this point we can start diving in and conquering the first dragon.

If you found you got most stressed out when trying to make decisions then skip down to the procrastination part of the behavioural section.

Work on the suggestions within that and record the improvements.

Now for some lucky people it will be that simple. But for most of us we will find that several things seem to conspire together to stress us out.

For us we need to take one step at a time. This means getting one reason under control then work on the next most important reason and then the one after that.

Please do not try and do several at the same time unless they are closely related.

If you feel that there are three or four equally critical but seemingly unrelated reasons causing you stress then pick whichever of these you wish and tackle it, then go to one of the others.

Now at this point you may well be saying to yourself "I can't handle this!" or "This is impossible!"

You are right of course they are, **if,** you convince yourself by using these types of phrases, because they increase your stress in a given situation *and* they stop you from searching for solutions.

Instead turn the statement into a question like "*How* can I handle this?" or "*How* is this possible?" this will open up your imagination to the new possibilities.

5 DEALING WITH ...MENTAL STRESS

Worry

Worry and anxiety can take over the life of some people.

What is worry, and what causes it?

Worry is an anxious state of mind brought about by over-concern with the future and fear about what it might bring.

At the heart of worry lies a preoccupation with unknown outcomes. Worry is often caused by a lack of acceptance of the fact that many outcomes in life cannot be controlled.

By repetitively casting about for solutions, worriers feel they are doing something to address their situation.

Worry can lead to problem-solving BUT only when it is done in a calm mental state that allows solutions to emerge. This is not always as easy as it sounds.

Self-help strategies include relaxation and meditation, exercise and practising the technique of structured problem solving.

Read through the suggestions below and then start using the the one with which you feel most comfortable.

Over night

A popular technique is to visualise the situation that is worrying you and visualise putting it in a pot, and putting a lid over it. Then put the pot on a back burner in your mind, and ask your subconscious to work on the problem overnight. Then forget about it and go to sleep!

In the morning, think about that situation and see if the mind overnight has cooked up a solution.

Quite often the solution will be there.

Your brain has been cooking up a solution whilst you were asleep.

To put it more flippantly...

"Hi brain, I've got a problem but I'm too screwed up to sort it out. So I'm going to sleep, you sort it out and tell me the answer in the morning."

If the problem is complex the solution may take a few nights to sort it out, each morning or evening you can refine the situation ready for the brain to cook up a few more suggestions.

Schedule Worry Time

One of the most effective techniques for worriers is to schedule a specific time of day for worrying, and to allow worried thoughts only during that time.

If you find yourself unable to stop worrying, allow yourself 10 minutes per day to worry.

Pick a regular time for this to occur.

When the time comes, set a timer for 10 minutes, and worry to your heart's content, writing down your concerns if it helps.

When the timer goes off, shift your attention away from worries, and tell yourself you can think about them again tomorrow at the same time.

This reassures the worried part of your mind that it will have a chance to go over the situation again, yet allows you to limit the amount of time spent worrying.

Focus on Solutions

When you're worrying, you're thinking about problems or potential challenges.

To stop worrying, try shifting to a problem-solving mode.

As soon as you notice your mind spiralling into worries, make a conscious effort to stop your circular thinking.

Then brainstorm a few possible solutions to the worrisome situation. Write them down if it helps you to focus.

In some cases, you may realise that you're not worried about anything in particular, but instead have a more general sense of "free-floating" anxiety.

If so, try one of the strategies below.

Structured problem solving

Structured problem solving is a method of turning fruitless worrying into strategies to find solutions.
It is best to practise first on small worries or problems, and limit yourself to working on one problem at a time.

As you become proficient at the technique, you can tackle larger, more complex problems.

You should write down all the steps.

The steps of structured problem solving include:
Step one – Identify the problem and be precise. For example, 'I am afraid of being alone in the house at night.'

Step two – Brainstorm every possible solution you can think of, without censoring any idea at this early stage. Give yourself permission to list even absurd or outlandish possibilities.

Step three – Evaluate the solutions one at a time, noting the advantages and disadvantages of each.

Step four – Decide on the most appropriate solution(s). It is sometimes better to choose a solution that can be implemented immediately, even though it might not be 'the best'.

Avoid choosing solutions that are too ambitious or hard to fulfil.

Step five – Make a plan for how you intend to implement the solution.
Include factors such as the required resources (like money), help required from other people, time limits or deadlines.

Possible difficulties that may be encountered along the way, coping strategies for those anticipated difficulties, rehearsal (like practising what to say during a job interview).

Methods of monitoring and reviewing the effectiveness of the plan.

Step six – Review the plan as necessary, perhaps adding or deleting points.

Other ideas for redirecting your worry include:

Imagine a stop sign in your mind each time a worry arises.

Use a rubber band around your wrist to flick as a gentle reminder not to let worrying take over.

Think of something positive, such as a loved one or a recent good experience, to shift your attention away from your worries.

By taking the time to practise these strategies, you'll find that you can take control of your worry before it controls you and in the process, you'll nip stress in the bud.

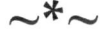

Anxiety

First
Release yourself from your symptoms.

When you have a surge of fear or anxiety, lie down and rest.

Don't act on impulse. Slow down.

Stop criticizing your partner / colleague and burdening them with your troubles.
When you begin to feel self-pity, don't indulge those feelings.

Turn to something else, like housework, mowing the lawn or even television.
If you feel like complaining or whining, stop yourself.

All these measures are like putting the brakes on a runaway car.
In this case, the mind is the car, and you can't stop it with one tap of the brakes.

You have to begin to gain some distance and clarity.
Imbalance makes that hard, but you must try.

Then
Take positive steps to regain balance.

Begin with a steady routine, however much you have avoided it in the past.

Go to bed at regular hours.
Eat meals on time.

Make sure you get out of bed only after you've had at least seven hours of sleep.

Provide yourself with a neat, reassuring environment.

Settle your mind, read books on healing, take time to walk every day, associate with calmer, more secure people.

Find a confidant you can trust to give you sound advice.

Stop associating with those who bring you down by making your situation seem hopeless, or whose problems only compound yours.

If possible, find a close friend who has compassion and can offer you kindness.

~*~

Perfectionism

Aiming for perfection in itself is not a bad thing.

However once you are obsessive about it then stress levels can increase dramatically.

Challenging Perfectionist Behaviours and Beliefs:

Step 1: Identify behaviours

Start by writing down everything you do that must be "perfect" – at work, in your home life, in your hobbies, and in your personal relationships.

For example, perhaps you check your work multiple times, or turn it in late because you worry you didn't do it correctly.

Perhaps you arrive at appointments very early, because you're afraid of being late.

Or you might spend an inordinate amount of time tidying up your desk; time that you could spend relaxing or working on other projects.

Also, examine things that you don't do, because of perfectionism.

Step 2: Identify Beliefs

Next to each behaviour, write down why you believe this action must be perfect.

For instance, imagine that you never delegate tasks to your assistant, even though this is why you hired him. You often stay late at work to finish tasks that he could have done.

You don't delegate tasks, because you believe he'll do them incorrectly, and you'll look bad.

Step 3: Challenge the behaviour.

Once you've done this, come up with one specific step to overcome each behaviour.

For instance, you could try delegating one non-urgent task to your assistant.
Once it's complete, review it once to make sure that he completed it correctly.

Or, if you check your work endlessly because you believe you may have made a mistake, resolve to read it over twice: once after you finish it, and once at the end of the day.

Step 4: Evaluate the Results

Once you successfully challenge the behaviour, look at what happened.

Chances are, there weren't any negative consequences.

So what did you learn?

Practice this regularly with different behaviours.

You'll likely experience some anxiety while challenging your perfectionist behaviours.

This is normal.
However, you'll probably find that your anxiety decreases dramatically once you see the results.

Tip:

Challenge just one behaviour at a time: trying to change all of your behaviours at once may cause you too much anxiety.

Other Strategies for Dealing with Perfectionism:

As well as the steps above, you can use these strategies to deal with perfectionism:

1. Set Realistic Goals

Perfectionists often set goals so high that there's little hope of achieving them.

Instead, learn how to set realistic goals. Come up with several lifetime goals and then break these down into yearly and monthly goals. It can feel great to achieve these smaller goals!

To start with, try setting daily realistic goals, then at the end of each day put a tick beside those you achieved.

If you did not achieve the majority then you are still setting unrealistic goals.

Once you can set realistic goals for daily targets, then start on the longer term ones, taking on board the new knowledge of what is realistic.

2. Listen to Your Emotions

Whenever you're feeling anxious, unhappy, or scared about a task, ask yourself whether you've set your goal too high. Your emotions may be telling you that you're trying to achieve an unrealistic goal.

If you catch yourself engaging in self-sabotage, such as telling yourself that you're not good enough, stop.

Remember that your thoughts influence your mood and, often, your actions.

Instead, focus on using positive statements about yourself and your abilities.

These statements can raise your self-esteem and reprogram your thinking.

Remember, you always have a choice in what you think and do.

3. Don't Fear Mistakes

Mistakes are part of life.

They can even provide rich learning experiences, if you have the courage to examine them.

Your mistakes can teach you far more about life and your abilities than your successes will.

Make a real effort to learn from each mistake that you make.
You'll grow as a result.

4. Readjust Your Personal Rules

Perfectionists often live by a rigid set of rules.

These rules could range from "I must never make mistakes" to "There must never be a crumb on the kitchen table."

Although it's healthy to have high personal standards, they need to be flexible and helpful, not unrelenting and unrealistic.

Identify one rule you live by that's rigid, unfair, or unhelpful. Then reword it to be more helpful, flexible, and forgiving.

For instance, imagine you never suggest new ideas during team brainstorming meetings, because there's never enough time to think them through.

You fear suggesting an idea that might make you look bad, so you always keep quiet.

Your personal rule is that you should never offer an idea until you've had plenty of time to perfect it.

You could readjust this rule by saying, "Ideas don't have to be perfect during brainstorming sessions.

The team's purpose is to take rough ideas, talk them through, and determine whether they're sound.

My team will appreciate my input."
Then put your new rule into practice!

5. Focus on the Whole

Perfectionists often exhibit "tunnel vision": they focus on one small part of something and ignore the rest.

For instance, if you're on a diet, you might obsess about slipping up and eating dessert at lunch, while ignoring the fact that you've stuck to your diet for the past three weeks.

Challenge this by making an effort to look at what you've done right.

Don't focus exclusively on the negative!

6. Watch What You Tell Yourself

Whenever you tell yourself that you "must," "should," or "shouldn't" do something, pay attention to how this demand makes you feel: perfectionists often use these words when they're setting up personal rules.

Some examples are "I must never make mistakes" or "I should have done that job instead of delegating it."

Be careful using these words in your thinking; they can often lead you to create unrealistic expectations.

7. Relax and Be More Spontaneous

Perfectionists often find it difficult to relax and be spontaneous.

Relaxation and spontaneity are not only necessary for a healthy life, but they can also improve your productivity and well-being.

Take regular breaks when you're at work to stretch, walk around, or do deep breathing exercises. Add spontaneity to your life by stopping to watch the sunset, or by picking up a new hobby.

Key Points

Perfectionism, in the form of "maladaptive perfectionism," can push you to set unrealistically high goals. It can also reduce productivity and creativity, and can lead to various health problems. To overcome your perfectionist behaviours, start by listing everything you do (or don't do) because of your desire for perfection.

Next, identify why you believe that each task has to be perfect, and come up with an action that you can take to challenge this behaviour.

Focus on one behaviour at a time – if you try to overcome several behaviours at once, it may leave you feeling stressed, which means that you're far more likely to quit.

Also, set realistic goals, listen to your emotions, and don't fear mistakes.

Become Aware of Your Tendencies

You may not realise how pervasive perfectionism can be.
By becoming more aware of your patterns, you're in a better position to alter them.

If you're able, it's a great idea to record your perfectionism thoughts as they pop into your head.

If it's impractical for you to jot thoughts down as they come, it's a great idea to go over your day each night.

Remember the times when you felt you'd failed, or hadn't done well enough, and write down what you thought at the time.

This will help you become more aware of perfectionism thoughts as they come to you in the future.

(You can even write a journal on your feelings about these thoughts, but don't feel you've 'failed' if you don't have time to do this!)

See the Positive

If you're struggling with perfectionism, you probably have honed the skill of spotting mistakes in even the best works of others and of yourself.

You may just naturally look for it, and notice it above all other things.

While this habit may be difficult to just stop, you can soften your tendency to notice the bad by making a conscious effort to notice all that is good with your work and the achievements of others.

If you notice something you don't like about yourself or your work, for example, look for five other qualities that you *do* like.

This will balance out your critical focus and become a positive new habit.

Alter Your Self-Talk

Those who wrestle with perfectionism tend to have a critical voice in their head telling them their work isn't good enough, they're not trying hard enough, and they're not good enough.

If you're going to overcome perfectionism, you need to work on changing this little voice!

Negative self talk can perpetuate unhealthy behaviours and wreak havoc on your self esteem.

By altering your self talk, you can go a long way toward enjoying life more and gaining an increased appreciation for yourself and your work.

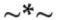

Long work hours

When job and workplace stress threatens to overwhelm you, there are simple steps you can take to regain control over yourself and the situation.

Good time management is essential for coping with the pressures of modern life without experiencing too much stress.

Good time management doesn't mean you do more work. It means you focus on the tasks that matter and will make a difference.

Whether it's in your job or your lifestyle as a whole, learning how to manage your time effectively will help you feel more relaxed, focused and in control.

If you never have enough time to finish your tasks, better time management will help you regain control of your day.

Here are some suggestions for reducing job stress by prioritising and organising your responsibilities.

Tasks can be classified in four simple ways to determine which should be done first through to those that can be delegated or ignored.

Time management

One   *It is important and urgent*

Your waste paper bin is on fire
Your flight to Berlin leaves in ten minutes

Two   *Important but not urgent*

Reading articles in relevant technical magazines
Go for a walk at lunchtime

Three   *Not important but urgent*

The ringing telephone or mobile
Looking at emails immediately they arrive

Four   *Not important not urgent*

Discussions on the variety of sandwiches you are
each eating.
Sending and reading silly emails.

Clearly anything that is important and urgent must
be done straight away.

After that what is it that as the day goes by builds
up the need for longer and longer work hours?

It is failing to deal with the important but not
urgent tasks

The key to reducing stress if you are overworked is to be able to plan ahead. You cannot do that whist you are wasting time on unimportant items, even if they try to claim that they are urgent.

Use voice mail to record phone messages and only listen to them when you have finished a task. Do not let them interfere with your schedule.

With emails, only look at them first thing in the morning, after lunch and just before you go home.

Reduce job stress by prioritising and organising

Once you start recognising and dealing with interruptions you will become more organised.

This sense of self-control will help you in stressful situations and will often be well-received by co-workers, managers, and subordinates alike.

This in turn can lead to better relationships at work.

Clearly this by itself will not eliminate all of the need to work long hours.

Consider the work you are doing, does it all need to be done by you?

Could you delegate it?

Quite often your co-workers appreciate rather than resent the extra work.

Now this next suggestion may seem counter-productive but please consider it seriously.

Have a lunch break

Many people work through their lunch break to gain an extra hour at work, but this can be counter-productive.

Make a point of taking at least 30 minutes away from your desk it; will help you to be more effective in the afternoon.

A break is an opportunity to relax and think of something other than work. Go for a walk outdoors or, better still, do some exercise.

Then when you come back to your desk you will be re-energised, with a new set of eyes and renewed focus.

Planning your day with a midday break will also help you to break up your work into more manageable chunks.

Most of us do not like getting up earlier than we have to. However, if you are currently arriving at work flustered and in a rush, consider the following.

Would you like to arrive at your place of work in a calm and relaxed state fit and ready for the day ahead?

Then all you need to do is start your journey 15 minutes earlier.

Getting to work before everyone else gives you the time to sort out your day before all the interruptions start.

Once you have taken all the above on board you should be ready to start actively scheduling your day and week.

Make a list

A good way to stay organised and take control of your projects and tasks is to use a to-do list to write things down.

The simplest of list is just that, its value is that every time you complete a task you put a big tick by it.

I prefer a two column list.

Put all the important items on the left column and everything else on the right column.
Only do those on the left. Only tackle anything on the right when the left column has been completed.

This can be refined by prioritising.
So once you have your list give each item a number where I is the most important, 2 the next and so on.

There are many variations so try a few and see what works best for you.

Keeping a list will help you work out your priorities and timings, so it can help you put off the non-urgent tasks.

This in essence is what is meant by working smarter, not harder.

Good time management at work means doing high-quality work, not high quantity.

Concentrate not on how busy you are but on results you can achieve.

Spending more time on something doesn't necessarily achieve more.

Staying an extra hour at work at the end of the day may not be the most effective way to manage your time.

Life style choice

If after doing or trying to do the above you find you are still stressed to breaking point, take a step back and ask yourself – am I in the right job?

We should be working to live, not living just to work.

6 DEALING WITH
PHYSICAL STRESS

Lack of sleep

Having the occasional restless night is one thing but when it persists then quite rightly something must be done to sort it out.

The environment

Take a look round the room you try to sleep in.

How can you eliminate the distractions and develop a calm environment?

Make sure the bed is comfortable, the coverings can be adjusted to keep you warm or cool depending on the time of year.

The room is quiet and dark, keep windows closed if there is a lot of traffic, if you need more air, open the door to the hallway.

Eliminate blinking lights from electronic gadgets.

Then close your eyes and go to sleep.

Not enough?

Then next stage is to consider what you are doing prior to preparing for sleep.

First try to get into a regular routine.

Get into bed at roughly the same time every evening.

Don't do anything like watching TV, playing video games, sending text messages, making phone calls.

Get the body used to this routine.

Next cut down on stimulants in the two hours prior to going to bed.

Stop drinking coffee, tea or alcohol and no cigarettes. (Don't panic, once the body has got back into a sleep pattern you can experiment with relaxing the rules).

All of this takes time, so what do you do when you are dog tired in the middle of the day?

A power nap of 20 minutes (no longer) in the afternoon (not morning) is the best solution, sure it may be hard to keep going but you do need to get the body back into a better routine.

This for most people will sort out the mechanical side but if the main problem is stress then other remedies are also required.

Read again the section on relaxation then check through the index to see what areas of stress you may be suffering and then follow the suggestions.

Always keep in mind, there is a solution but it may take perseverance to find it.

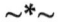

Travel

So how exactly do you beat the perils of travel-related stress?

Essentially, much of the stress incurred by travelling has to do with simple worries: missing your plane or forgetting vital documents, such as passports or currency.
This is easy to conquer if you take positive action and prepare in advance.

Plan Ahead

I am preparing a detailed book covering all types of transport and all causes of travel stress. For this book I am concentrating on flying and vacations.

It is easy to forget this one, but it cuts out a lot of stress if dealt with.

Are all the people in your group comfortable with the plan, are you all looking forward to it?

If not then get those issues sorted before going any further.

So if everyone is happy with the destination then planning the travel could be the key to a brilliant vacation.

Check that all passports are valid and cover the time you will be away, plus any overlap time the country demands.

If the journey is fairly short and is just from A to B then you can probably do it all   the planning yourself online.

However if you are planning multi flights and or moving from location to location then strongly consider using a travel agent preferably one you can speak to face to face.

Whatever your choice travel early in the day, earlier flights are less likely to be delayed.

Much as we might all like to travel first class, reality is that we will probably end up in tourist, but this can still be great.

With the possible exception of some budget no frills airlines you can pre-book your seats.

Make sure you do that and do it at the earliest possible time. Also get as near as you can to the front. I will explain why later.

And do print out your boarding cards at home if possible and do the return journey as well.

All these little things reduce the stress level at the airport.

Right, you have your flights and accommodation sorted, you all know the why, when, where and how so you can now use the Internet to research the area you are going to visit.

This will help remove the worry of what are the right clothes to wear and take.

It will also help in deciding what medication is easily available and what you need take to take with you.

Now start a list(s).
Put on it all the things that worry you and tick them off as you resolve them.

Packing
Get organised well in advance.

Decide between you now to be either a max or min.

There is not much point in one of you going for the minimum and just having cabin luggage if the rest have to book in suitcases.

Have a list for each member of the family.

Be aware of the weight restrictions and don't bother to pack up to the limit, you will need some spare weight for the extras you buy whilst you are away.

Make a list of all the things you may need to bring with you, and check them off as you pack them to better ensure that you don't leave behind things you'll need.

Pack the night before you leave, or earlier, to avoid the stress of being rushed.

It also gives you the opportunity to remember and pack things you may otherwise forget.

Keep things you may need at the ready while in transit in your carry-on bag, but stow the rest of your items in your checked luggage to reduce your chances of getting held up at security points.

Jabs

If you are advised that the place you are going to suggests you have certain vaccinations - have them. One less thing to get stressed out on whilst you are away.

Travel insurance may or may not be a waste of time, but if you have got it then you will not worry quite so much if anything goes wrong.

So that's it - Nothing to get stressed up about...

Remember what we said right at the beginning of section 2.

If there is something (anything) that is upsetting you, do something about it.

If there really is nothing YOU can do about it, accept it and get on with the rest your life.

You have done the preparation, you have your lists so stop being stressed about preparation.

Now whilst you cannot do anything yourself about

weather, strikes, war etc., you can be up to date with the various situations.

Stay abreast of delays by checking your airline's website a week or so before you go, be aware of the method they like to be contacted and if you have any worries contact them or your travel agent.

It is always not knowing that causes stress, once you know the cause you can better appreciate the situation.

Before you leaving home check for delays, this may save you avoid spending hours sitting in a waiting room.

Airports' websites are useful too, as they can inform you of security measures that are in place ahead of time so you can plan for them.

Plan your journey to the airport just like everything else, well in advance.

Allowing yourself ample time before your flight can reduce some of the stress of finding parking, checking bags, moving through security, and other aspects of travel that are much more stressful when you're rushed.

If you end up being early, you can read a book, listen to music, or take a walk through the airport and get some exercise before you leave.

If you get held up in the process of getting to your

plane, at least you won't then have to spend energy worrying about missing your flight.

There will be a degree of waiting around. It is a fact of life so accept it and don't let it get under your skin.

If you are travelling as a family group, a pack of cards can be a useful distraction.

If you are on your own, make sure you have your Kindle or a good book.

Security

There will be a queue.

The earlier you join it the better. If you leave it to the last moment you will get all stressed up that you may miss your flight.

You wont miss your flight because some harassed check-in attendant will be looking and calling through the queues to find and fast track you.

But you will still get stressed.

So at the earliest time, start your trek through security.

If you have done your preparation correctly you will not have any sharp objects or prohibited substances so no need to get stressed over that.

Make sure you have put all your metal objects (like keys) in your carry-on bag rather than your pockets. Then you won't have to empty your pockets of them as you pass through the airport metal detector.

Wear your rose coloured spectacles and let all the noise, pushing and shoving pass over and around you. There is nothing you can do other than endure it so accept it as one of life's necessities.

Departure lounge

When your flight is called, don't immediately rush into the queue.
Stay sitting calmly reading or whatever.

Let the bulk of the passengers struggle onto the plane, then when calmness has returned stroll down and onto the plane.

Remember you have a reserved seat so there is no need to sit an extra 10 minutes on a noisy hot plane.

Arrival at your destination.

About 20 minutes before landing pay a visit to the facilities (get there just before the last minute rush).

Once the plane has landed the benefit of having a seat near the front will become obvious.

You will be amongst the first off the plane, thus

you will also be amongst the first to get through immigration.

You have now arrived and your stress level is almost normal, congratulations.

To sum it all up – it is all about having the right attitude.

Rather than thinking of all this as a stressful hassle, think of it as an adventure or at the very least, a challenge.

With the right attitude (and thorough preparations), travelling can be fun and not at all stressful.

The majority of travel-related stress can be beaten simply by remaining calm and composed.

Make sure you keep your head above water when travelling and, if adverse events do occur, simply tackle them one step at a time.

As a result, you'll find that your holiday will get off to a much more relaxing start - a trend that can only continue into your vacation.

~*~

Stress ~ manual labour

Whether you are a construction worker, a mechanic, or a factory worker, blue collar job stress can have an effect on your physical, mental, and emotional health.

While working at a physically demanding job, you'll be using more energy so balancing the amount of energy (food) you put in is important.

A high-quality, healthy diet is not only essential for building resilience, but also for maintaining health. If you have a poor quality, junk food-filled diet, then you will get exhausted earlier and this will build up your stress levels.

Ideally you need to get in the habit of eating at least one gram of animal protein per pound of bodyweight, plenty of healthy fats and sufficient vitamins and minerals every 3 hours.

Don't panic, I appreciate you cannot have a lunch break every 3 hours.

Here is a solution.

Liquids – Just liquefy meat or fish and a selection of grain, potato, vegetables and cheese. You will need to experiment to get a palatable taste. A quick search on Google should find a good range of recipes.

So get the blender out and start making nutritious concoctions which you can take to work with you in a flask. Then you can have quality nutrition every three hours with minimal hassle.

This probably wont stop you going home tired but you shouldn't be exhausted.

This in turn will give your brain the energy to help you relax and take the stresses out of the day.

Worry

Worry builds up the stress levels.

The worry and stress may be be due to your opinion of management decisions (or lack of them) and the impact it may have on future employment.

If there are ways you can make suggestions in a non confront-able way then try them, if not shrug your shoulders and stop worrying.

In the meantime keep your ear to the ground for other job openings where prospects are better.

It is a fact of life that it is easier to change jobs than to get one if you are out of work.

Hobbies

The other big area is to cut off work completely once you leave the premises.

The best way to do this is to have a hobby that you can completely immerse yourself within.

So find something, anything that will interest you and join a local club for that subject.

Very soon you will find that you can cut your mind off from work.

7   DEALING WITH
   EMOTIONAL STRESS

Sadness & depression

Identifying Your Kind of Sadness

It's perfectly normal to have sadness in your life. Some kinds, however, can be a cause for concern.

If you are feeling sad at this moment or have been experiencing a down mood for a while look honestly at your situation.

There are three types of sadness most of us fall into:

Short-term sadness
 This is a passing mood, lasting a few days or, at most, a week. It sometimes has a cause and sometimes not.

The best remedy is to lower your stress by going to bed early and get eight hours of uninterrupted sleep.

Also take on some exercise and break up your normal routine a bit.

Boredom, lack of sleep, being too sedentary are all associated with sad moods.

Triggered sadness

This includes a downturn in mood because something undeniably bad has happened to you, such as losing your job or the death of someone close to you.

In such a situation, you will generally know what the trigger is.

The problem is that most people feel helpless when they enter extended sadness, even when they know there is a good reason for it.

In this case, you need time to process your sadness, let nature take its course and try to share your feelings with other people.

Bottling up your feelings and feeling victimised is never helpful.

Triggered sadness lasts a period of time, in an emotionally healthy adult, within six months there

is a return to the level of emotions that existed
before   the   trigger   was   set   off.

Depression

If you feel sad, exhausted, helpless, hopeless and
unable to sleep, eat or enjoy sex for a period of time
lasting more than a few weeks, you should suspect
that you are depressed.

There is often a trigger for this condition, but it is
usually something that you could normally cope
with.

When coping breaks down, depression takes over.

So if you feel that you can't cope, even with minor
stress and ordinary setbacks, mild to moderate
depression may be indicated.

This is a complicated mood disorder that varies
from person to person.
If you suspect that you or someone close to you is
depressed, a visit to your doctor is needed.

Tackling sadness

Sadness like a lot of other stresses can feel infinite
in its affects on your life. So the first thing to do is
to try and corral it.

Get a lined note pad. Draw a line all the way down
the middle.

Next write down every single negative thought that enters your head.

Include everything that's bothering you.

Anything at all that is bothering you, even an untidy room, a waste paper bin that's full to overflowing, a split nail, everything, just put it on the list.

Once that is done, feel within yourself that you have accomplished something, you have your demons out in the open.

Now comes the really exciting part.

We are going to look at that list, sure it may be several pages long but we are going to tackle everything on there and find a solution to all of them.

Start at the top with the easy ones those that can be dealt with straight away, if you feel sadness or depression rising on a particular item skip past it.

Do just the things that you can like finding a nail file or scissors and trimming the nail, or emptying the waste paper basket and put a big tick in the right hand column.

Do it straight away then move on down the list.

Sure it may take a couple of days but just doing this easy bit will lighten your load.

Once you have done that you will find some on the list that you skipped past a little easier to deal with. So do those.

Then we are left with the harder ones

In all probability the ones left are expressed in a negative fashion, for instance you may have written "I have no friends".

So in the right hand column write down all the people you come in contact with daily or weekly, then cross off the list those who you definitely dislike.

You will be surprised just how many are left. These are the core of your friends.

If you feel that you are not close enough to them then reflect on the type of conversations you have.

Just maybe they are all 'doom and gloom' and 'how hard done by' type of conversations.

So try being more positive: discuss what is good about life.

So for every negative write a positive in the right hand column. Keep working at the list every day and things will get better.

Apply this positive approach to all the items left on the list and amaze yourself as to how many ticks you are getting.

Be realistic

We do live in a society where a high value is placed on being positive.

Yet sometimes this simply isn't possible, and people find themselves facing temporary or long-term sadness.

Just telling yourself to "be positive" isn't much help, because moods can have a life of their own.

One of the pitfalls of positivity is that people tend to fantasize about a perfect life instead of realistically facing the fact that no life is perfect.

We all face challenges, disappointments, frustration and failed expectations.

So what can happen is that we become passive.

We distract ourselves by watching more television or spending more hours on the computer.

We wait for sadness to pass and we behave as if nothing bad is going on.
Keeping up a good front is important in most people's lives, yet behind the facade can lurk a good deal of fear.

Instead of positivity, what's needed is <u>reality</u>.

Being realistic means that you drop the main defence that all of us are tempted to employ - **denial**.

The only reason to deny your sadness is if you feel that you can't do anything about it.

But as we have shown there are concrete ways to cope with sadness and gain control over it.

So be realistic about your life: take this opportunity to relieve the pressures around you and lift the fog of sadness.

It may surprise you but, in fact, the best cure for sadness is happiness.

Anything that diminishes your ability to build your own happiness must be avoided or eliminated.

For example, don't hitch your happiness to external rewards or postpone being happy until sometime in the future.

Don't expect someone else to make you happy. Don't allow your emotions to become habitual and stuck or close yourself off from new experiences.

Don't ignore the signals of inner tension and conflict, dwell on the past or live in fear of the future.

Most of all: don't equate happiness with momentary pleasure.

Discover how to build a sense of happiness that no one can take away from you.

The journey to such happiness takes a long time, yet every step is one of fulfilment.

Loneliness

First of all, please don't feel you are weak or weird because you feel lonely.

There's no need to feel ashamed of your loneliness.

In fact, if you find one or two friends to talk with about it, you will probably find that they feel lonely also (or have at one time or another), and you can encourage each other.

Expect the best.

Lonely people often expect rejection, so instead focus on positive thoughts and attitudes in your social relationships.

One thing is certain: we cannot wish our way out of loneliness. Nor can we escape it by wishing others would change - either by gossiping about them, or by sedating ourselves with alcohol, frantic activity, and other excesses.

Here are some constructive ways to begin to deal with loneliness:

Slow down to be more attentive to yourself and your surroundings. This can begin by eating more conscientiously, making healthier choices and taking time to enjoy your food.

It might also mean scheduling regular walks or bike rides and stopping to notice some interesting shop or garden along the way.

Get a dog/cat to occupy you will help you from being alone. Playing with your pet also will reduce your stress.

Take up a new hobby.

Do something that you enjoy doing like painting, reading, and playing snooker. Maybe you can try some adventures sport like mountain climbing, jungle tracking, hunting and so on.

Browse through a museum, zoo or art gallery.
Study the night sky or visit a planetarium
Trace your family tree
Chart your horoscope

By keeping your mind occupied by visualizing positive affirmation you can overcome loneliness.

Finding any activity which can excite you whenever you are lonely will help towards reducing that feeling of loneliness.

Given time it will also introduce you to more people.

Experiment with new things in life - approaching a daily life in different perspective and doing the daily routine in different way is a good way to overcome loneliness.

Listening to your favourite music and recalling your sweet old memories also is a good way to overcome loneliness.

Join on-line communities like facebook, twitter or myspace. Getting introduced with different kind of people from all over the world and sharing your life with these new people will give a new meaning to a lonely life.

Call your friends and go out with your friends.

Get involved in the activity that you enjoy doing with your friends.

Feeling lonely is a state of mind. You can change it by just getting out of the situation.

A simple walk can rejuvenated you again.

Attend a country fair or community event.

Give your plants some tender loving care.

Visit a place of worship.

Take a bubble bath.

Cook your favourite meal.

Call a phone-in radio show; tap into a computer chat line.

Write a letter to the editor.

Ask yourself: "Am I falling into the trap of all work and no play?"

If so, consider setting goals in the following areas:

Personal well-being (physical / intellectual / spiritual).

Community activities.

Relationships (enhancing existing ones/forming new ones).

Send the Right Signals to People

Too often, we send people mixed social messages.

How many of us really mean, "Let's get together some time." We make dates, then cancel - "something came up."

Sending no messages will present yet another problem - when we wait for others to call us and when they don't, we write them off.

If you want to spend time with people, make the first move. Ask someone to join you for lunch or coffee, then schedule a time and stick to it.

Start being proactive

Develop a plan.

Whenever you begin to feel lonely do something.

Here are three suggestions:

Pick up the phone and call someone. Send a card to someone.

Visit someone—especially those who may be housebound or in a nursing home.

By taking your mind off of yourself and onto others, you will soon realize how very beneficial it is.

Stimulate Your Sense of Curiosity.

This is another way to move away from the feeling of loneliness.

Pick up a newspaper and look for an interesting event or function.

Consider attending as a curious observer rather than with the expectation that it must be fun or the perfect activity for you.

See what you can get out of it.

Perhaps, rekindle an old hobby by exploring what the new developments are. For example, the hobby of model railways has developed dramatically over the years.

Curiosity engages the mind. It encourages us to make connections, and seek answers. Certainly, it can help us strike up interesting conversations.

Consider Honing Your Social Skills

For some people, loneliness stems from not knowing the "appropriate" things to do or say socially. If you are concerned about this, check out the local book store or library for guides on etiquette, interpersonal relationships, and communicating.

One way to perfect your speaking skills is by joining Toastmasters International or a local equivalent.

Follow Your Interests

Enrol in an adult education course, attend antique shows or science fairs or organize an after-work event (such as a car rally or softball game) among your co-workers.

Some of the best friendships have been established through contact with other people that you share a common interest.

Reach Out As a Volunteer

Few activities bring such a sense of personal satisfaction and the feeling of being connected, than by providing a useful service for those needing it.

There are many possibilities - hospitals, animal shelters, recreation centres or a senior's facility, just to name a few.

Try "Reconnecting" With People

This could mean calling, writing or tracking down

old friends, former colleagues, and others you have lost touch with.

A relationship might flourish on having a meal together once a month, a letter or card several times a year, or a real gab session when one or both of you truly need it!

Doing things that get you to feel more "connected" can make all the difference in the world when it comes to dealing with loneliness.

You've just read some very good suggestions - many are planned social activities that involve others, like signing up for classes or community events.

Some of the suggestions do help with learning how to deal with the time you spend by yourself, as in finding enjoyment pursuing hobbies and interests.

Life is short. So we have to make sure we enjoyed every bit of it. There is no time for loneliness. Let's make our life a more interesting one.

Before we leave this subject let us look at the following;

What Is the Difference in Being Lonely and being Alone

Lots of relaxation, creative thinking and personal accomplishments are achieved on a solitary basis. If you are accustomed to being in the constant company of others, the appreciation of being alone may take some time and effort to develop.

Once you have told yourself it is okay, experiment with it and see if you can feel fulfilled on your own. Have fun indulging yourself in something you wouldn't do if others were with you.

Some people may find that they don't tolerate time spent alone well. If so, ask yourself "Do I just like being with others more or is there something I am afraid of when I am alone?"

If this is the case, it will help to identify the fear and then make a plan to solve the problem.

Some common fears are the fear of being bored and not being able to entertain; fear of feeling sad or depressed; fear of not marrying or having children in the future; and existential fears such as being alone in the universe.

How Much Time Spent Alone is Normal?

There is no correct amount of time to spend with people vs. being alone.

College students often experience many changes in personal contact levels that come with the other changes of being a student; a higher level of independence and choices in daily schedules, different living conditions and expanded opportunities for jobs and extracurricular activities.

With so many choices to make, some students find their days are filled with people. Some may find that without the built-in contact of high school peers and family, their paths rarely cross with others in any meaningful way.

Guilt

Everyone experiences guilt at one time or another during their life. While some guilt can induce positive change, it can also become self-destructive, wasting energy and adding stress to your life.

Read on for some tips on processing these feelings so that you can eliminate, or at least minimize, your guilt.

Identify whether or not you *should* feel guilty

Remember that guilt is evidence of a troubled conscience and, in some circumstances, is appropriate.

If, after careful thought, you conclude that your actions were wrong and that your guilt is justified, think of ways to make amends or make the situation "right."

Take action sooner than later to combat another emotion commonly associated with guilt: Shame.

Engage in self-exploration to really get in touch with your feelings

Explore your feelings on a deeper level to ensure that it is indeed guilt you are feeling.

When we feel guilty, we focus intently on events that have already happened.

When we worry, it is about events that are presently happening or may happen in the future. If it is worry, go to the earlier section on how to eliminate worry.

Affirm that the event has happened and that you feel guilty

Write it down if it helps.

Here are some examples:
"I let the dog out and he got run over by a car. I feel guilty that Bruno is now dead because we all loved him so much."

"I failed my driving test. I feel guilty that I let my parents down who paid so much for me to go to learn."

"I broke up with Mary. I feel guilty that he hurts so much."

Ask yourself, "Is there anything I can do to make this situation better right now?"

Here are some examples:

"There is nothing I can do to bring Bruno back, but you can apologize to all those who loved him so much, and you can learn from your mistake."

"I can study the theory paper more thoroughly and

concentrate more when on driving lessons."

"I could get back together with Mary, but that would be a short-term solution, since I would not be happy and we would end up in the same place. I could console her, but that will probably make the situation worse. I have exhausted all possibilities and there is nothing I can do to make this situation better."

Modify your behaviour so that it will not happen again

Write it down if it helps.

Here are some examples:

"From now on, I will check to make sure the gate is locked every time I enter and exit the garden so that if we get another dog, he will not escape.

"From now on, I will study as hard as I need to before my test so that I do well."

"Mary is too clingy and sensitive. From now on, I will not date girls like that because it will end badly just like this relationship did."

If you still feel guilty, affirm that it is not necessary or productive

Say to yourself, "I have now done everything in my power to make this situation better. My guilt no longer serves any positive purpose."

Move on with your life

Don't dwell on negative, guilty feelings; they lead to inappropriate levels of shame and self-loathing.

Recognize that nobody's perfect and we all make mistakes, and this is one you will not repeat.

Engage in activities that are positive and affirming, and where you have opportunities to do good; allow yourself to see how the same mistake that made you feel guilty has now resulted in your being a better, more conscientious person.

Guilt and Debt

We all have monthly bills that just have to be paid. Then whatever is left is what we have for household items, food and entertainment.

It is all too easy to become guilty by spending some of this money on simple pleasures for ourselves. It feels as though we are depriving others within the family.

If this is you then you need to step back and look at the bigger picture. None of us can live constantly on bread alone. From time to time we do each need a break from the challenges of day to day living.

So build this into your monthly plan, let it be an open part of your budget.

Take a hard look at your budget — and build in some spending on yourself.

Track your spending for a month, then take a look at the necessities (your rent or mortgage, utilities, and savings) and the non essential items and decide where you can cut back.

If you can, set aside money to spend on "extras" like entertainment, outings, shopping, and so on. That way, you'll feel justified spending money on yourself because it's already planned.

It's easier to spend on yourself when you don't feel like you're stealing from Peter to pay Paul.

Talk it through with your spouse or partner.

Talk about your feelings regarding spending, and make sure both of you are involved in the nitty-gritty of your finances. That means paying bills together, balancing the credit card each month, and going over bank statements.

If you don't normally handle the bills, getting involved will help relieve some of your anxiety about financial issues. And if you usually take care of the accounting, your partner will get a better sense of the family budget.

Make sure you and your partner agree on how to spend any money that's left over each month after paying the bills. That way, no one feels like they're being cheated.

~*~

Anger

The moment a feeling of anger starts to arise is the time to employ this simple exercise adapted from the HeartMath Go to Neutral Tool.

- Take a time-out to disengage from your thoughts and feelings, especially stressful ones. Actually say to yourself, "time out," as you recognize and feel your emotional triggers, then step back from all reactions to them.
- Shift your focus to the area around your heart and feel your breath coming in through your heart and going out through your solar plexus.
- Tell yourself, "Go to neutral," then remain in this neutral zone until your emotions ease and your perceptions relax.

Angry Thoughts;

"He is looking over here at me and thinks I'm stupid"
"They always let me down"
"She just doesn't care about me, she is selfish"

Write down some of your thoughts now and write as many answers or balanced thoughts as you can.

The aim is to get faster at catching these "hot thoughts" when they come into your head and answering back straight away. It takes a lot of practice but really does work.

Myths

Here are some examples of these unhelpful beliefs and ideas on how to challenge and question them.

I can't control my anger, my father was angry and it is something I inherited from him.

This is the idea that anger is something you can't change – it's in your make up, something you were born with. It is an excuse, that lets you off the hook in terms of controlling your anger.

We know that some people are born with tendencies to be more emotional, fearful, angry or sad.

The way we react to these emotions however is learned, and we can tackle our own angry behaviour by changing the way we respond to events and people.

If I don't let my anger out I'll explode

It has long been a popular belief that some emotions and drives build up, like steam in a pressure cooker and need some way out or else they become harmful.

If you hold this point of view losing your temper could be seen as something healthy. But we know from research that people are often left feeling much worse after losing control of anger.

Shouting, hitting, slamming doors can all increase and strengthen feelings of anger.

If you don't show anger you're either a saint or a wimp

This is an example of black and white thinking. You think that if you're not angry and aggressive then you're a hopeless wimp.

But the best way to deal with a situations, is not to be angry and out of control, but to be firm, sure and in control – to be assertive.

My anger is something people fear and it stops them taking advantage of me

This belief sees anger as a protector and other people as dangerous.
It may be that this belief was correct at a particular time of your life, but if you continue to think this way, it can cause problems.

Good friendships are not formed on fear and you will be unlikely to have good friendships and relationships because of your angry behaviour.

It is also likely to backfire, where others with problems of anger will see you as threatening and possibly pick fights with you.

If I get angry it takes my anxiety away

This belief is often found in people who have been the victims of violence or aggression. It is better to try and tackle your anxiety by other ways rather than exchanging one unpleasant emotion for another.

Anxiety can only be overcome by facing what you fear and finding ways of overcoming it.

I have good reason to be angry because of things other people have done to me

Anger is a natural reaction when we are mistreated or taken advantage of. But if this anger continues into all areas of your life then it will cause difficulties for you.

If the mistreatment took place a long time ago and the people who did it are no longer in your life it may help to ask "where does this anger get me now?"

In summary
We need to look carefully at the angry "hot thoughts" we have and try to see if we are making errors in the way we view situations.

It can help to try and have more balanced thoughts.

We also need to examine long held beliefs about our anger and challenge those, which are unhelpful.

Remember, logic can defeat anger!

Controlling the physical symptoms of anger

Relaxation and calming methods can help to reduce angry feelings.

If you are with a partner who also becomes angry it may help if you both learn these relaxation techniques.

You need to learn to use the following approaches automatically if you are in a difficult situation.

Reducing physical symptoms

In order to reduce the severity of physical symptoms it is useful to "nip them in the bud", by recognising the early signs of tension and anger.

Once you have noticed early signs of tension you can prevent anger becoming too severe by using relaxation techniques.

Some people can relax through exercise, listening to music, watching TV, or reading a book. Picturing a pleasant scene in your mind can also help.

For others it is more helpful to have a set of exercises to follow.

Some people might find relaxation or yoga classes most helpful, others find tapes useful.

You can obtain a relaxation disc from your GP, and there are also a wide number of relaxation discs available in the shops.

A booklet available in this series also describes how to use relaxation.
Remember relaxation is a skill like any other and takes time to learn.

Keep a note of how angry you feel before and after relaxation, rating your anger 1-10.

Controlling breathing

It is very common when someone becomes angry for changes to occur in their breathing.

They can begin to gulp air, thinking that they are going to suffocate, or can begin to breath really quickly.

This is called over-breathing, it has the effect of making them feel dizzy and therefore more tense. It can lead to unpleasant feelings but is not dangerous.

Try to recognise if you are doing this and slow your breathing down.

Getting into a regular rhythm of "in two-three and out two-three" will soon return your breathing to normal.

Some people find it helpful to use the second hand of a watch to time their breathing.

Controlling angry behaviours

If we look back to the vicious circle of anger, it becomes clear that if we can challenge our angry thoughts and reduce the physical symptoms of anger then we should not get to the point where we begin to behave angrily.

No-one is perfect however!

If we do not manage the previous stages it helps to have ideas on how to tackle the angry behaviours we might normally show.

We can do this in three stages:

Stage 1
Be very clear what your angry behaviours are – what comes before them and what happens afterwards. It can help to keep a diary over a short period to help you understand this.

Before my anger; Initial thoughts and feelings; Behaviour; What happened afterwards

For example, 'Alex' continually 'blows his top' in

home, work and social situations, he has tried to understand this by keeping a diary of what happens on these occasions.

Stage 2
Make a list of all the other things you can do instead of behaving angrily.
When you have done this choose the best new approach(es) to try in difficult situations.
Here is 'Alex's' list as an example.

1 Excuse myself and leave the situation for a minute, "I'll be back in a minute", return when calmer.

2 Take a deep breath and relax self for a second.

3 Ask the other person to let me know why they have said something, try and understand them.

Ask, "Why do you want me to let you know when I'll be in?,"
"Why do you say our section is doing less?"

4 Ask the other person to sit down and talk about it. Say, "Let's get a cup of tea and talk about it ..."

Stage 3
Try to adopt the new behaviour in situations where you feel angry. Keep a diary of how it went.

Helpful ideas for changing angry behaviours can be:

Timing – if you tend to get angry at certain times when you talk to someone eg at night, try and talk to them calmly at different times of the day.

If particular things make you angry – it may be you can avoid them, eg don't travel to the shops when you know you'll get stuck in traffic for ages.

Use a quick relaxation and/or breathing exercise.

If you hate to sit in when your partner watches sport, plan something else at that time.

If you hate his friend don't be around when the friend is there.

Count to ten before responding.

Go for a quick walk.

Ask yourself at this time "Why is this making me angry?"

Ask yourself at this time, "Is this worth getting angry about?"

Use calming self statements in your head, eg "calm down", "getting mad won't help", "just forget it".

In summary

In order to control angry behaviours you need to:
Know what your angry behaviours are.

Decide what other behaviours might take the place of your angry behaviour.

Try out these new behaviours

Problem Solving

Sometimes real worries and stress can make us more irritable and angry. A problem solving approach may help in this.

A good way to begin is to write down a problem. Describe it as clearly as you can, for example "I never have any money", is too vague, something like "I owe 3000 to different credit card companies", is more helpful.

Next, write down as many possible solutions as you can. It doesn't matter how silly you may think the solutions are, the point is to think of as many as you can.

Try to think how you have solved similar problems in the past.
Ask a friend what they might do.
Think to yourself what you might advise a friend to do if they had the same problems, eg possible solutions:

Get all debts on one loan with less interest.
Agree on affordable payments.
See a debt counsellor.
Get a part time job.
Sell car.

Choose what seems like the best solution and write down all the steps it would take to achieve the solution.

Who might help?, what might go wrong?, often it is helpful to think "what is the worst thing that could happen?".

If you can think of a plan to cope with this, your anxiety might reduce.

If you are trying to come up with a plan to tackle a problem that has been worrying you for some time, it is often helpful to discuss this with a friend or even your doctor.

Stressful lifestyle may lead to anger.

Nowadays life is often stressful, and it is easy for pressures to build up.

We can't always control the stress that comes from outside but we can find ways to reduce the pressure we put on ourselves.

Try to identify situations you find stressful by noticing the beginnings of tension.

Take steps to tackle what it is about these situations that you find stressful.

~*~

Fear

What's the worst that could really happen?
Everything we tend to worry about seems really silly doesn't it?
Worry about grades...traffic....a report for work....what people think of you....our retirement funds...etc.

How are these even comparable to real life-threatening situations?

How can someone living in a war-torn country have less stress than someone sitting in an office typing on a computer?

How can people who seem so poor on the outside have no stress and an abundance of happiness....yet someone with a big house and bank account is unhappy and stressed out all the time?

Why are movie stars with nothing to worry about all turning to drugs and alcohol?

Something isn't right here, we need real perspective to help us out. Time to step back and look at our lives from a distance....like you were watching some tv show and you were the main star.

You can plan, you can study, you can save money...but to worry about things that have yet to happen or may never is really a waste of energy.

We do this to ourselves too....no one is forcing us to worry, it's all us.

Worry, doubts and fears are all based on things that have not happened....and not what you need to do right now.

Really...will most of the stuff you worry about on a daily basis even matter in a year? Will anything you worry about even happen at all??

Probably not.

Whatever it is that scares you, here are 10 ways to help you cope with your fear and anxiety:

1. Take time out

It feels impossible to think clearly when you're flooded with fear or anxiety. A racing heart, sweating palms and feeling panicky and confused are the result of adrenalin. So, the first thing to do is take time out so you can physically calm down.

Distract yourself from the worry for 15 minutes by walking around the block, making a cup of tea or having a bath. When you've physically calmed down, you'll feel better able to decide on the best way to cope.

2. What's the worst that can happen?

When you're anxious about something, be it work, a relationship or an exam, it can help to think through what the worst end result could be. Even if a presentation, a call or a conversation goes horribly wrong, chances are that you and the world will survive.

Sometimes the worst that can happen is a panic attack.

If you start to get a faster heartbeat or sweating palms, the best thing is not to fight it.

Stay where you are and simply feel the panic without trying to distract yourself. Placing the palm of your hand on your stomach and breathing slowly and deeply (no more than 12 breaths a minute) helps soothe the body.

It may take up to an hour, but eventually the panic will go away on its own. The goal is to help the mind get used to coping with panic, which takes the fear of fear away.

3. Expose yourself to the fear

Avoiding fears only makes them scarier. If you

panic one day getting into a lift, it's best to get back into a lift the next day. Stand in the lift and feel the fear until it goes away. Whatever your fear, if you face it, it should start to fade.

4. Welcome the worst

Each time fears are embraced, it makes them easier to cope with the next time they strike, until in the end they are no longer a problem. Try imagining the worst thing that can happen – perhaps it's panicking and having a heart attack. Then try to think yourself into having a heart attack.

It's just not possible. The fear will run away the more you chase it.

5. Get real

Fears tend to be much worse than reality.

Often, people who have been attacked can't help thinking they're going to be attacked again every time they walk down a dark alley. But the chance that an attack will happen again is actually very low.

Similarly, people sometimes tell themselves they're a failure because they blush when they feel self-conscious. This then makes them more upset.

But blushing in stressful situations is normal. By remembering this, the anxiety goes away.

6. Don't expect perfection

Black-and-white perfectionist thinking such as, "If I'm not the best mum in the world, I'm a failure," or, "My DVDs aren't all facing in the same direction, so my life is a mess," are unrealistic and only set us up for anxiety.

Life is full of stresses, yet many of us feel that our lives must be perfect. Bad days and setbacks will always happen, and it's essential to remember that life is messy.

7. Visualise

Take a moment to close your eyes and imagine a place of safety and calm: it could be a picture of you walking on a beautiful beach, or snuggled up in bed with the cat next to you or a happy memory from childhood. Let the positive feelings soothe you until you feel more relaxed.

8. Talk about it

Sharing fears takes away a lot of their scariness. If you can't talk to a partner, friend or family member, call a helpline such the Samaritans (08457 90 90 90, open 24 hours a day). And if your fears aren't going away, ask your GP for help. GPs can refer people for counselling, psychotherapy or on-line help through an on-line service.

9. Go back to basics

A good sleep, a wholesome meal and a walk are often the best cures for anxiety. The easiest way to fall asleep when worries are spiralling through the mind can be to stop trying to nod off.

Instead, try to stay awake.

Many people turn to alcohol or drugs to self-treat anxiety, with the idea that it will make them feel better, but these only make nervousness worse. On the other hand, eating well will make you feel great physically and mentally.

10. Reward yourself

Finally, give yourself a treat. When you've picked up that spider or made that call you've been dreading, reinforce your success by treating yourself to a candlelit bath, a massage, a country walk, a concert, a meal out, a book, a DVD or whatever little gift makes you happy.

The fear of flying can spoil a holiday before it has even begun. If this is a fear you have then read and believe.

Top Tips for fearful flyers.

Have confidence that, despite all your feelings, flying is normal.

Although you may not believe it, flying an airliner is NOT complicated or difficult.

Flying and safety is most definitely NOT in the hands of chance or the Gods.

Aircraft don't mind being in cloud, even dark cloud.

Planes do not defy the laws of gravity.

Flying is safe because of the laws of physics and gravity.

Remember, flying is much safer than you think.

Remember that the fear of flying is a learned fear and therefore it can be unlearned.

'What if ' thoughts must be controlled.

The fear of flying is not a weakness.

Be content with small steps.

Praise your achievements.

Planes don't plummet... they descend.

The pilots know what they're doing.

You don't need to hang on to the armrests.

Aircraft make a lot of noise while taking off.

Turbulence is uncomfortable but that's not the same as dangerous.

Let the airline know that you are an anxious flyer when you buy your ticket.

Eat lightly; salads and watery fruit are ideal.

Get good quality sleep before your flight.

Put your seatbelt on as tightly as you can bear it.

There are no such things as air pockets.

An aircraft will not fall out of the sky if the engines stop.

An airliner can glide for over 120miles from cruising height.

'Stalling' has nothing to do with the engines.

There are no 'dangerous' airports to land at.

Aircraft do not fly through thunderstorms. They have to stay 20 miles away.

Aircraft on commercial flights do not turn lower than 500 feet above the ground.

Clear air turbulence is no worse than any other turbulence.

In reality it's unlikely that you have experienced severe turbulence.

Being struck by lightning in an aircraft will not hurt you or the plane

What's abnormal, unusual or unexpected to you...is normal to the pilots and crew.

Remember aircraft are more efficient than birds...birds don't carry passengers.

An aircraft would glide 'if' the engines stopped.

The engines are not straining on take off.

"Flying is safer than you think"

If you are still not satisfied - See more at: http://www.flyingwithoutfear.com/

8 DEALING WITH... PSYCHOLOGICAL STRESSES

How Can You Manage Marriage Stress in Troubling Times?

Marriage is the unconditional love for your partner.

As you read through this section please keep this in mind and refer back to it.

It is not a specifically 21st century problem but something that has been around for centuries. But this is of little consequence when you are stressed out with difficulties be it that you are married or just living together.

If solutions were easy then there would be no divorce, so what can be done?

Even when you believe your partner is completely in the wrong keep on offering unconditional love.

Just as important is communication.

Find a way to be able to express your views without indicating blame.

Be prepared to shoulder the blame even when you think you are not at fault.

None of this relieves the stress level but it is the essential first stage.

As in times gone by, it is frequently the lack of money that is the cause of disputes and unhappiness.

It is very easy to believe your partner is spending too much and you are the only one making an effort to cut back.

So once again a list is called for.

Start making a list of all money coming in and all money being spent.

Sure you will have a big gap where you seem to have money left over as far as your list is concerned but in reality that 'spare' money does not exist.

Next at a time when you are both relaxed and are not about to rush off somewhere explain to your partner what you have been doing.

Ask what it is that you have forgotten to add to the list.

Try and get a dialogue going without implying fault.

At some point you will need to decide just what to cut back on, ask for suggestions, offer suggestions and not just ones for your partner to do.

The very act of doing this will mean you are working together against the wicked world rather than against each other.

Weathering the storms together

Any of the following can create high stress levels in a marriage:

Financial troubles, unemployment, intimacy problems, infidelity, differing views on parenting, chronically poor health of a dependent family member, the death of a child and clashes with in-laws.

Each can be resolved more easily if you are open and talk through the issues, without portioning out blame.

Work through the easiest first and gradually work up to the big one.

Remember you are a partnership vowed to help each other in times of hardship.

Dealing with stress in relationships is often frustrating and difficult. Sometimes, we get it all wrong and make matters worse.

There are some steps that we all can take when coping with stress in relationships and reducing the stress that naturally comes with those dilemmas.

Here are just a few:

Identify the problem
You can't solve a problem if you don't know the particulars. What type of trouble, very specifically, are you experiencing in a troubled relationship? When you answer that question, you can begin to work on it in a positive way.

Avoid the water-boarding effect
Some people experience a "water-boarding" effect within their relationships. That occurs when constant arguments, physical or emotional abuse, criticism or other problems are experienced – not on a daily basis, perhaps – but are constantly on your mind and wreak havoc with your emotions.

Avoiding the issues will only continue to bring stress into your life, so it's imperative that you address these problems either with the other person or with a relationship expert.

Stop second-guessing

You can't read minds – and neither can anyone else. Don't try to second-guess what's going wrong in your relationship and causing stress.

Blaming yourself or the other person exclusively isn't productive – nor is it likely to be true. It's imperative that you address specific actions or words that are causing the problems and then work on solving them.

Identify external negative forces

Are finances, work, other relationships, dishonesty or deception causing problems in an important relationship?

Think about this carefully and if possible, discuss it with the other person. It may be possible for the two of you to find solutions by talking it out or seeking outside help.

Take control of yourself

You can't make a person love you, care for you, treat you with respect or anything else you may desire.

You can only control how you react to these problems. Don't keep beating your head against a wall – realize that you and only you are in control of your life.

Get help

There is so much help for troubled relationships in the form of books, life coaches, counsellors, religious institutions and even on-line help. Seek help to solve the problems and reduce the stress in your relationship.

Sometimes we lose our balance and perspective, we can't see the forest for the trees and may need a boost to our thinking powers. There is help available. Get the help you need!

Whittling away at the problems that lurk in a relationship will likely produce results.

But, if nothing seems to work and you're in an abusive relationship or one that's causing such stress that it's affecting you both physically and mentally, concentrate instead on becoming the person you want to be.

There's a beautiful person that lies within you that the universe is waiting to meet!

Financial or career pressures

If your finances are getting out of hand, it's time to take more control over them. Conversely, if you're too controlling over your money issues, perhaps it's time to let loose a little.

Financial stress can stem from many different situations.

Try and identify what is causing the stress and then consciously work towards eliminating it from your life.

Debt:

If your bills are piling up and you don't know where to begin, start by seeking professional help. Yes, it's hard to face the reality of your financial situation, but living a life of uncertainty and angst is not going to work.

The sooner you address the problem head on the better you'll feel. The longer you put it off, the more damage you'll inflict on yourself emotionally, mentally and physically.

To successfully cope with your pressures, you need to recognize what demands are being placed on you that are making you and your body behave this way.

Once you do that, figure out if those demands and expectations are realistic and achievable.

If they're not, re-assess your goals to something that is more reasonable. If your demands are realistic, identify why you aren't meeting those expectations. Sometimes dealing with stress is as simple as being more accountable.

Getting your finances in tune is always going to be a crucial part of achieving your goals.

There are four basics to revamping your financial life:

Stick to a budget, cut expenses, reduce debt and start saving.

Setting your budget in the simplest terms can be done on one sheet of paper.

Put your income at the top of the page, and from that number you deduct your expenses. The amount left over is what you can spend on other things, such as reducing debt and increasing savings.

Having a written budget gives you confidence in your personal financial strategy, which can help you dramatically lower your financial stress level.

Our goals are frequently linked to our careers.

Career:

Do remember, we control our career, our current employer is only there to help us achieve it.

If your current employment is causing you to daily get more and more stressed, then it is time to step back and examine your personal objectives.

Do you enjoy working to deadlines?

If you don't but your current job demands it then it is time to change.

Be assured it is always easier to get another job whist employed than when you are unemployed.

Do you like the process of decision making but are stuck in a job where all the decisions are made by others?

Consider the option of starting your own business.

Quite frequently we find ourselves promoted from a doer of tasks to managing others. This usually gives us an increase in salary but can massively increase our stress levels.

If this happens <u>get some specific training</u> related to what you are now doing, even if you have to pay for it yourself.

Earlier chapters cover many of the stresses that the working day brings up. So if you have jumped straight to this section then at a suitable time read through some of the other relevant chapters.

Finally, and most importantly, find time to rest, relax and exercise.

Your life is a giant combination of many aspects. Take a break from financial concerns.

Go for a jog or a picnic in the park with family. You'll be healthier and both activities will help you relax.

Don't let one negative area dominate everything else.

Carve some time out of your day to enjoy doing the things you love doing.

Be sure you find time to enjoy the finer things in life.

After all, it's only money.

~*~

Challenges with life goals, and general state of happiness

We all have dreams as to what we want to achieve in life.

So, if as life develops we find ourselves drifting away from the dream future, we panic.

Stress builds up and we begin to wonder what life was all about.

Now is the time to wake up from the dreams and make some realistic decisions on what you want from the rest of your life.

Start by deciding on five things you want to have done in ten years time.

It could be visit a rain forest, own your first motor car, buy a house, get your children through university.

It can be anything that is <u>measurable</u>.

Now with each of these work backwards with what you need to do to achieve these goals.

Let's use buying a house as an example.

Most of us will need a loan for the bulk of the purchase and find the difference between the full price and the loan from our savings. If the buying price is 200,000 and we have to raise 40,000 from our own savings then we need a plan.

By year five we need to have in savings 15,000 and be saving 5,000 each year to reach our target of 40,000.

By year three we need to have established a regular means of saving 500 every month.

By the end of year one you need to have the first 1,000 safely tucked away in your savings account.

By the end of the first six months you need to have stopped buying unnecessary objects of desire and put that money into your savings account.

This week you will open a savings bank account and start putting all your spare money into it.

The above is very simplistic but it shows you how to focus on a desirable long term dream.

If you have five of these, they do not all need to be financial.

You will be able watch their progress, have a purpose in life and see your dreams being fulfilled.

Your stress levels have been converted into pleasures.

Beware of setting your targets too high or unrealistic. Planning to marry a Prince is one thing, planning to marry a future King of England would not be so realistic!

Once you have established the realistic things in life that you can and want to achieve then your stress levels will calm down. You will also find yourself to be a happier person.

Happiness comes from being satisfied with the way your life is developing.

It is enhanced by seeing to good things that are happening around you.

It is going out each day and trying to find at least one good thing that has happened, rather than moaning about all the bad things around you.

Remember what was said at the beginning of section two?

If there is something (anything) that is upsetting you, do something about it.

If there really is nothing <u>YOU</u> can do about it, accept it and get on with the rest your life.

9 DEALING WITH
A COMBINATION

Very few of us have just one simple cause for stress.

If you can determine the major cause then start with that, otherwise start at the top and work your way through.

Recognising your stress triggers

If you're not sure what's causing your stress, keep a diary and make a note of stressful episodes for two to four weeks. Then review it to spot the triggers.

Things you might want to write down include:

- The date, time and place of a stressful episode
- What you were doing.
- Who you were with
- How you felt emotionally.
- What you were thinking.
- What you started doing.
- How you felt physically.

A stress rating (0-10 where 10 is the most stressed you could ever feel)

You can use the diary to:

Work out what triggers your stress
Work out how you operate under pressure
Develop better coping mechanisms

Doctors sometimes recommend keeping a stress diary to help patients diagnose stress.

Am I in control of stress or is stress controlling me?

- When I feel agitated, do I know how to quickly calm and soothe myself?
- Can I easily let go of my anger?
- Can I turn to others at work to help me calm down and feel better?
- When I come home at night, do I walk in the door feeling alert and relaxed?
- Am I sometimes distracted or moody?

- Am I able to recognize upsets that others seem to be experiencing?
- Do I easily turn to friends or family members for a calming influence?
- When my energy is low, do I know how to boost it?

Take action to tackle stress

There's no quick-fix cure for stress, and no single method will work for everyone.

However, there are simple things you can do to change the common life problems that can cause stress or make stress a problem.

These include relaxation techniques, exercise and talking the issues through.

What else can I do?

Have more fun
Schedule in and actively pursue activities that you enjoy and that help you relax.

Express your feelings
Unexpressed emotions are the building blocks of pain and illness, so give vent to your emotions.

Get enough sleep
Poor sleep habits interfere with your body's ability to rest, heal and recharge. If you have trouble sleeping, seek out the causes and get some help addressing them!

Exercise

Regular physical exercise is one of the best ways to clear away tension and build energy. It also helps you to adopt a better life perspective and to feel more in control of your circumstances.

Practice relaxation exercises

Breathing, meditation and visualization exercises help you let go of mental worries and allow you to experience precious moments of calm and inner peace.

I believe that this quiet, "nothing happening" space is where the healing process begins.

Develop good relationships

It is important to have genuine friends in whom you can confide and find support. Those who love and accept you, people who will listen and advise but won't judge are your true friends. It can also be very fulfilling to be a true friend to someone else.

Experience love and satisfying sex

If you currently have a primary relationship that's loving, sensual and sexual in your life, it can be a major stress reducer.

Change perceptions and attitudes

When ideas or views are not serving you, it's wise to examine and adapt them.

It's important to learn to respond to life's situations and not just react.

Hanging onto frustrations, holding grudges, and playing the victim/blame game are not in your health's best interest.

Eat right.

Eating nutrient-poor foods that are high in sugar or filled with chemicals and unhealthy fats puts an unnecessary stress on your system, reducing your immunity, overloading your liver and forcing your body to work overtime just to maintain balance.

Eating nourishing food supports your body's natural immune and healing systems, helping your body to cope successfully with other sources of stress.

Managing stress in daily life

Stress is not an illness itself, but it can cause serious illness if it isn't addressed. It's important to recognise the symptoms of stress early.

Recognising the signs and symptoms of stress will help you figure out ways of coping and save you from adopting unhealthy coping methods, such as drinking or smoking.

Spotting the early signs of stress will also help prevent it getting worse and potentially causing serious complications, such as high blood pressure.

There is little you can do to prevent stress, but there are many things you can do to manage stress more effectively, such as learning how to relax, taking regular exercise and adopting good time-management techniques.

10   WHEN TO SEE YOUR GP

If you've tried self-help techniques and they aren't working, you should go to see your GP. They may suggest other coping techniques for you to try or recommend some form of counselling or cognitive behavioural therapy.

If your stress is causing serious health problems, such as high blood pressure, you may need to take medication or further tests.

Mental health issues, including stress, anxiety and depression, are the reason for one in five visits to a GP.

Get stress support

Because talking through the issues is one of the key ways to tackle stress, you may find it useful to attend a stress management groups or class.

These are sometimes run in doctors' surgeries or community centres. The classes help people identify the cause of their stress and develop effective coping techniques.

Ask your doctor_for more information if you're interested in attending a stress support group. You can also use the search directory to find emotional support services in your area.

AND FINALLY

I do hope this book has been of some help to you.

I am planning to go into even greater depth on some of the sub-headings.

If you wish to be kept up to date on the progress of them or anything else related to stress please email me at qualityman@quality-solutions.co.uk

Please tell your friends, pass on the title and author by every means you can. The more we can do to help people reduce their stress levels the happier they will be.

Also a review on Amazon would be very much appreciated.

Thank you,
John Harriyott

Further reading:

The following Amazon books may be of interest.

How to Master Anxiety by Joe Griffin & Ivan Tyrrel

How To Stop Worrying and Start Living by Dale Carnegie

Control Stress by Paul Mackenna

How to Achieve Stress-free Productivity by David Allen

ABOUT THE AUTHOR

John is a well travelled Englishman.

He is married has two sons and two grandchildren.

His career has been engineering based and he rose through the ranks to the highest level.

For the last 20 years he has run his own consultancy business, specialising in quality improvements for small businesses.

Over the years with specialist training, personal experience and insights gained whist travelling, John has built a store of knowledge which he has now started to share.

This is his first venture into publishing.